THE
COMPLETE
DIABETIC
COOKBOOK:

Delicious and Balanced Recipes Made Easy

By
CHARLIE MASON

TABLE OF CONTENTS

As promised, please use your link below to claim your 3 FREE Cookbooks on Health, Fitness & Dieting Instantly

https://bit.ly/2MZF09w

You can also share your link with your friends and families whom you think that can benefit from the cookbooks or you can forward them the link as a gift!

INTRODUCTION

Congratulations on purchasing this book and thank you for doing so.

The following chapters will discuss recipes that make it easy to enjoy food while also keeping your blood sugar levels in balance. This ensures that you are able to eat many of your favorite foods without causing your blood sugar levels to spike.

With this diabetic cookbook and the included diabetes recipes, you will find it easy to prepare a wealth of quick healthy and delicious meals for any time of the day. Whether you have Type 1 or 2 diabetes, this diabetic cookbook makes sure that you are never feeling deprived of the foods that you love most. It also makes it easy to get creative which is something missing from many other diabetic cookbooks and meal plans on the market.

You will first learn about the breakfast recipes so that you can start your day right. From there, get delicious recipes for lunch and dinner, as well as a wealth of snacks to keep you satiated in between meals. The diabetic cookbook desserts included allow you to indulge your sweet tooth without the glucose spike or guilt.

Many diabetic diets tell you that sweets and convenience foods are completely off the menu. However, it does not have to be this way. Instead, you simply make a few quick changes to the preparation process and ingredients. You still get to enjoy the same decadent flavors so that food can still be a very enjoyable part of your life. Remember that just because something is healthy does not mean that it has to be boring or without great flavor. With a little creativity and a few small changes, your favorite foods stay on the menu and continue to taste great.

For example, for breakfast, your chai latte and an omelet are easy and enjoyable. For lunch, fill up with a quick and easy Mediterranean turkey wrap or summer chicken spring rolls. For dinner, baked red snapper or lime and garlic grilled clams give you an elegant dinner favorite. Get decadent for dessert with peanut butter swirl chocolate brownies or a slice of homemade coconut cream pie. In between meals, snack on garlic herb parmesan dipping sticks or a sweet and spicy snack mix.

There is no need to be a chef or spend hours in the kitchen to enjoy great food that is nutritious, delicious and filling. Think about the foods you love the most and look at the recipes here to try something new or to enjoy an old favorite with a healthy twist.

There are plenty of books on this subject on the market, thanks again for choosing this one! Every effort was made to ensure it is full of as much useful information as possible, please enjoy!

CHAPTER 1

DIABETIC-FRIENDLY BREAKFAST RECIPES

It is important to eat a healthy breakfast, but mornings can be tough and rushed. These quick and easy recipes make it possible to enjoy a great breakfast every day without it causing you to be late. Each breakfast recipe can be prepared from start to finish in no more than 15 minutes. Much of the preparation can even be tackled the night before to reduce the overall preparation and cooking time.

Chai Latte

This recipe makes 1 serving and takes approximately 8 minutes to make.

The 1 chai latte contains:

Protein: 4 grams

Fat: 2 grams (0 grams saturated fat)

Sodium: 61 milligrams

Cholesterol: 10 milligrams

What's in it

- Ground cloves 0.125 teaspoons

- Vanilla extract 0.25 teaspoons

- Sugar substitute 2 packets

- Orange spice tea 0.5 cups

- Warm 2 percent milk 0.5 cups

How it's Made

1. Brew the tea until it reaches the desired strength, with greater strength being ideal for this drink.

2. Put the ground cloves, sugar substitute and vanilla extract into the desired cup or mug.

3. Pour in the milk.

4. Pour in the brewed tea.

5. Stir the contents until fully blended.

Mushroom, Broccoli, and Cheddar Omelet

This recipe makes 2 servings and takes approximately 15 minutes to make.

1 serving contains:

Protein: 18 grams

Fat: 7 grams (2.4 grams saturated fat)

Sodium: 530 milligrams

Cholesterol: 190 milligrams

What's in it

- Reduced fat cheddar cheese 1.5 tablespoons
- Nonstick cooking spray
- Thawed, frozen broccoli 1 cup
- Sliced mushrooms 0.5 cups
- Chopped onion 0.25 cups
- Extra virgin olive oil 0.5 teaspoons
- Freshly ground pepper 0.125 teaspoons
- Egg whites 4
- Whole eggs 2

How it's made

1. Put the egg whites and whole eggs in a bowl and whisk together until light in color and fully combined. Add the pepper and whisk until it is mixed in well.

2. In a medium saute pan, spray the nonstick spray and pour in the olive oil.

3. Put the mushrooms and onions into the pan and cook until softened. Add the broccoli and heat thoroughly.

4. Remove the vegetables from the pan and spray more nonstick spray. Pour in the egg and egg white mixture. Cook until the eggs are nearly set.

5. Pour the vegetables into the egg toward the center. Apply the cheddar cheese.

6. Fold the egg over and cook it until the cheese is melted and eggs are completely d1.

Pink Grapefruit and Avocado Salad

This recipe makes 8 servings and takes approximately 10 minutes to make.

1 serving contains:

Protein: 1 gram

Fat: 3.5 grams (1 gram saturated fat)

Sodium: 50 milligrams

Cholesterol: 0 milligrams

What's in it

- Salt and pepper to taste
- Cilantro, leaves only, 4 sprigs
- Pink grapefruit 1
- Avocado 3

How it's made

1. Peel, pit and chop the avocado into bite sizes.
2. Peel and cut the grapefruit into bite sizes.
3. Place the avocado and grapefruit into a bowl.
4. Season with salt and pepper.
5. Garnish with sprigs of cilantro.

Fresh Basil and Sausage Frittata

This recipe makes 4 servings and takes approximately 15 minutes to make.

1 serving contains:

Protein: 21 grams

Fat: 8 grams (2.4 grams saturated fat)

Sodium: 525 milligrams

Cholesterol: 50 milligrams

What's in it

- Fresh basil 0.25 cups
- Tomatoes 1 cup
- Green onion 0.5 cups
- Part-skim shredded mozzarella cheese 1 ounce
- Egg substitute 1.5 cups
- Chicken sausage 8 ounces
- Extra virgin olive oil 2 teaspoons

How it's made

1. Pour the olive oil into a pan set over medium heat.
2. Place the sausage into the pan and cook until it starts to brown, flipping it as needed.

3. Pour the egg substitute into the pan, allowing it to evenly spread over the sausage, and cook for approximately 1 minute and then remove from the heat.

4. Place the green onions, basil, cheese, and tomatoes on top and evenly.

5. Cook until cheese melts and egg substitute is thoroughly cooked.

Baked Egg and Avocado Salad

This recipe makes 2 servings and takes approximately 15 minutes to make.

1 serving contains:

Protein: 8 grams

Fat: 8 grams (2.5 grams saturated fat)

Sodium: 80 milligrams

Cholesterol: 185 milligrams

What's in it

- Chopped cilantro 0.25 cups
- Thinly sliced and peeled red onion 2 ounces
- Thinly sliced large tomato 1
- Cubed avocado 2 ounces
- Cracked black pepper 0.5 teaspoons
- Kosher salt 1 teaspoon
- Fresh lime juice 1 fluid ounce
- Canola oil 2 teaspoons divided
- Whole eggs 2

How it's made

1. At 400 degrees Fahrenheit, preheat the oven.

2. Crack the eggs, ensuring the yolks are not broken, into their own bowl.

3. Preheat a small pan that is safe for the oven and pour in 1 teaspoon of canola oil. Carefully put the eggs into the pan and place it into the oven. Cook these for approximately 2 to 5 minutes.

4. Grab a small bowl and combine 1 teaspoon of canola oil, salt and pepper and lime juice. Whisk these ingredients together until they are completely mixed.

5. Add the tomato, cilantro, avocado and red onion to the dressing mix and toss until they are fully coated.

6. Place the salad mix in a place and then carefully place a cooked egg on top of each avocado.

Green Smoothie Breakfast Bowl

This recipe makes 2 servings and takes approximately 10 minutes to make.

Each serving contains:

Protein: 11 grams

Fat: 10 grams(0.9 grams saturated fat)

Sodium: 180 milligrams

Cholesterol: 5 milligrams

What's in it

- Toasted almonds and coconut mixture 1.4 ounces
- Frozen, sliced banana 1 medium
- Baby spinach 2 cups
- Frozen mixed fruit 1 cup
- Greek yogurt, fat-free, 4 ounces
- Unsweetened almond milk 0.75 cups

How it's made

1. Combine all of the ingredients, except the toasted almonds and coconut, into a blender.

2. Use the puree setting to mix all ingredients until they are the desired thickness. Add a little more of the unsweetened almond milk to make it thinner if this is desired.

3. Pour the mixture into 2 bowls, both containing equal amounts, and then top with approximately 0.5 ounces of a mix of toasted almonds and coconut.

CHAPTER 2

DIABETIC-FRIENDLY LUNCH RECIPES

About 4 to 5 hours following breakfast, it is common for the stomach to start grumbling, ready for another meal. Most people have 30 to 60 minutes for lunch, so time is of the essence. However, you need something that is going to satiate you while being tasty and nutritious. These lunch choices can be made relatively quickly, and you can even make them the day before and quickly reheat them for lunch for a delicious and filling meal.

Skillet Tortilla Pizza

This recipe makes 4 servings and takes approximately 15 minutes to make.

Each serving contains:

Protein: 5 grams

Fat: 3.5 grams (1.3 grams saturated fat)

Sodium: 290 milligrams

Cholesterol: 10 milligrams

What's in it

- Part-skim shredded mozzarella cheese 1 ounce
- Chopped fresh basil 0.25 cups
- Sliced green bell pepper 0.25 cups
- Sliced red onion 0.25 cups
- Sliced turkey pepperoni 0.5 ounces
- Dried pepper flakes 0.125 teaspoons
- Pizza sauce 0.25 cups
- 10-inch flour tortilla 1

How it's made

1. Grab a frying pan that accommodates the tortilla, coat it with cooking spray and heat the tortilla for 2 minutes over medium heat. Respray the pan, flip the tortilla and repeat.

2. Once the tortilla is flipped, put the sauce on the cooked side, ensuring that it is spread evenly.

3. Place the remainder of the ingredients onto the sauced tortilla in the desired order but place the cheese last.

4. Allow the cheese to melt by covering the pan with the appropriate lid.

5. Cut the pizza into 4 even slices.

Mediterranean Turkey Wrap

This recipe makes 4 servings and takes approximately 10 minutes to make.

Each serving contains:

Protein: 36 grams

Fat: 7 grams (1.6 grams of saturated fat)

Sodium: 605 milligrams

Cholesterol: 55 milligrams

What's in it

- Diced green olives 4
- Reduced-fat crumbled feta cheese 0.25 cups
- Diced Roma tomatoes 1 cup
- Diced and peeled cucumber 2 large
- No-salt-added turkey 12 ounces
- Heated whole-wheat wraps 4
- Hummus 8 tablespoons

How it's made

1. On each heated whole-wheat wrap, evenly spread 2 tablespoons of hummus.

2. Place 3 ounces of turkey onto the hummus. Put 0.25 cups each of diced cucumber and tomatoes. Add the diced olive and 1 tablespoon of feta cheese.

3. Carefully fold the wrap until it is cylindrical and the desired thickness.

4. Repeat this for the other 3 wraps.

Greens and Beans Soup

This recipe makes 2 servings and takes approximately 20 minutes to make.

Each serving contains:

Protein: 14 grams

Fat: 6 grams (0.9 grams saturated fat)

Sodium: 235 milligrams

Cholesterol: 0 milligrams

What's in it

- No-salt-added white beans, rinsed and drained, 0.66 cups

- Ground nutmeg 0.125 teaspoons

- Cayenne 0.125 teaspoons

- Crumbled dried marjoram 0.25 teaspoons

- Snipped fresh parsley 2 tablespoons

- Chicken broth with no fat and limited sodium 1 cup

- Undrained, no-salt-added sliced tomatoes 14.5 ounces

- Thawed and squeezed, chopped and frozen spinach 10 ounces

- Finely chopped celery 0.5 medium rib

- Finely sliced green onions 3 small

- Olive oil 2 teaspoons

How it's made

1. Heat the olive oil after placing a pan over medium heat. Make sure to maneuver the pan so that it is evenly coated.

2. Put the celery and green onions into the pan and cook for approximately 5 minutes so that they are tender but still crisp.

3. Add the spinach to the pan and cook for approximately 3 minutes. Stir frequently.

4. Add all other ingredients, except the beans, and take the heat up to medium-high. Cover the ingredients and allow them to come to a boil. Once boiling, let the ingredients to simmer at a lower heat while still covered for about 10 minutes.

5. Add the beans to the mixture, and without the cover, cook for about 1 minute so that the beans get heated completely.

6. Cook for an additional 8 to 10 minutes, partially covered, until the liquid has evaporated.

Pumpkin Risotto

This recipe makes 10 servings and takes approximately 30 minutes to make.

Each serving contains:

Protein: 11 milligrams

Fat: 3 grams (0 grams saturated fat)

Sodium: 230 milligrams

Cholesterol: 10 milligrams

What's in it

- Low-fat yogurt 2 tablespoons
- Grated Parmigiano-Reggiano cheese 4 ounces
- Vegetable stock 6 cups
- White wine 1 cup
- Finely chopped fresh pumpkin 1.25 pounds
- Carnaroli rice 2 cups
- Minced yellow onion 1 small
- Olive oil 3 tablespoons

How it's made

1. Grab a saucepan with a heavy bottom and place it on medium heat.

2. Warm the oil until it is hot, put the onion in and cook until it is tender, but make sure that it does not become brown. This takes approximately 3 to 5 minutes.

3. Add the pumpkin and the rice and stir. After about 30 seconds, pour the white wine and cook until all of the wine has evaporated.

4. Cover the rice with cooking stock, but only use enough to cover it. Once it is almost absorbed, add more. Keep doing this until all stock has been poured into the saucepan and the rice has absorbed it. This takes approximately 18 minutes.

5. Take the pan off of the stove and add the yogurt and cheese. Mix this well until the dish has a creamy texture.

Summer Chicken Spring Rolls

This recipe makes 4 servings and takes about 20 minutes to make.

Each serving contains:

Protein: 23 grams

Fat: 9 grams (2 grams saturated fat)

Sodium: 430 milligrams

Cholesterol: 60 milligrams

What's in it

- Medium spring roll skins 8
- Chopped green onion 1
- Sliced shiitake mushrooms 0.5 cups
- Chopped cilantro 0.25 cups
- Seeded, diced and peeled cucumber 0.5 cups
- Cooked and shredded chicken 2 cups
- Shredded cabbage 1 cup

Dipping Sauce Ingredients

1. Ground ginger 1 teaspoon
2. Olive oil 1 tablespoon
3. Hot water 2 tablespoons

4. Vinegar (rice wine) 3 tablespoons

5. Soy sauce (light option) 2 tablespoons

How it's made

1. Combine the chicken, cilantro, green onion, cabbage, cucumbers and mushrooms into a medium bowl.

2. For 10 to 15 seconds, soak each roll skin in water. Take approximately 0.33 cups of the vegetable and chicken mixture into the rolls.

3. Fold over the nearest edge so that it covers the filling. Repeat on the other side. Roll it outward and then seal it. Do this for all rolls.

4. To create the dipping sauce, put all of the ingredients in a container and whisk until completely blended together.

CHAPTER 3

DIABETIC-FRIENDLY DINNER RECIPES

After a long day, a nice dinner to relax and kill hunger is important. However, you are tired, and you do not want to spend hours coming up with a healthy dish. These dinner recipes are not overly time-consuming, and they have plenty of flavors. This ensures that you are getting important nutrients, filling your belly and getting a dish that is thoroughly enjoyable.

Mushroom and Walnut Meat Loaf

This recipe makes 4 servings and takes approximately 45 minutes to make.

Each serving contains:

Protein: 13 grams

Fat: 15 grams (2 grams saturated fat)

Sodium: 340 milligrams

Cholesterol: 45 milligrams

What's in it

- Finely chopped walnuts 0.5 cups

- Fat-free milk 0.5 cups

- Panko breadcrumbs 1 cup

- Beaten egg 1

- Freshly ground black pepper 0.25 teaspoons

- Sea salt 0.5 teaspoons

- Italian seasoning 1 teaspoon

- Rehydrated, minced sundried tomatoes 0.33 cups

- Diced red bell pepper 0.33 cups

- Finely chopped mixed mushrooms 1 pound

- Chopped onion 1 large

- Olive oil 1 tablespoon

- Cooking spray

How it's made

1. Preheat the oven to 350 degrees Fahrenheit.

2. Take 4 ramekins that hold 8 ounces and coat them with a nonstick spray.

3. In a pan, add the oil and then put it on medium heat.

4. Add the onions and mushrooms, and cook them for 10 minutes until they are browned.

5. Stir in the sundried tomatoes and red pepper, saute for about 8 minutes.

6. Add the salt and pepper and Italian seasoning. Saute for 1 more minute.

7. Take the mushroom mixture and put it into a large bowl. Let it sit for about 2 minutes so that it is able to cool.

8. Add the breadcrumbs, walnuts, milk, and egg. Gently mix all of these together and then evenly divide it into the individual ramekins. Press down so that the mixture is even with the top of the ramekin.

9. Grab a baking sheet and place the ramekins on top. Let it cook for 30 to 35 minutes after putting it into the oven.

Classic Beef Stew

This recipe makes 6 servings and takes approximately 2 hours to make.

Each serving contains:

Protein: 25 grams

Fat: 7 grams (1.5 grams saturated fat)

Sodium: 290 milligrams

Cholesterol: 45 milligrams

What's in it

- Freshly ground black pepper 0.25 to 0.5 teaspoons to taste

- Vinegar (red wine) 1 tablespoon

- Minced thyme 1 tablespoon fresh

- Frozen peas 1 cup

- Peeled carrots 3 medium

- Russet potatoes 2 large

- Minced garlic cloves 3

- Coarsely chopped onion 1 large

- Low-fat, reduced-sodium chicken broth 4 cups divided

- Cleaned, quartered and steamed cremini mushrooms 1.5 pounds

- Cubed top round 2 pounds

- Olive oil 3 tablespoons

- Seasoning (Italian) 1 tablespoon

- Whole-wheat pastry flour 2 tablespoons

How it's made

1. Combine the Italian season and flour in a container.

2. In a Dutch oven, use medium heat for the olive oil.

3. Coat the beef cubes in the flour and Italian seasoning and then brown in the Dutch oven.

4. Deglaze the pan after removing the browned beef cubes. Pour in 0.25 cups of chicken broth and the mushrooms. Sauté these until they are browned.

5. Deglaze the pan after removing the mushrooms. Pour in 0.25 cups of broth. Toss in the garlic and onions. Allow these to sauté for about 4 minutes.

6. Place the beef back into the pot and pour in the rest of the broth. Allow this to come to a boil. Once boiling, cover it and allow it to simmer for 45 minutes on low heat. Stir occasionally.

7. Toss in the potatoes and carrots. Let all of this cook for about 45 additional minutes.

8. Toss in the peas, red wine vinegar, mushrooms, thyme and black pepper. Mix all ingredients thoroughly.

Dijon Broccoli and Chicken with Noodles

This recipe makes 5 servings and takes approximately 35 minutes to make.

Each serving contains:

Protein: 36 grams

Fat: 7 grams (1.5 grams saturated fat)

Sodium: 150 milligrams

Cholesterol: 100 milligrams

What's in it

- Low-sodium Dijon mustard 3 tablespoons
- Fat-free, plain Greek yogurt 16 ounces
- Minced garlic cloves 2
- Onion 1 cup chopped
- Sliced mushrooms 8 ounces
- Olive oil 2 teaspoons divided
- Chicken tenders (all fat removed) 1 pound
- Cayenne 0.125 teaspoons
- Smoked paprika 1 teaspoon
- All-purpose flour 3 tablespoons
- Chopped broccoli florets 2.5 cups

- No-yolk, whole-gram noodles 6 ounces

How it's made

1. Follow the instructions on the pasta to prepare it, but do not add any salt.

2. About 3 minutes before they are d1, add the broccoli.

3. Drain the broccoli and noodles in a colander and set to the side.

4. Take a shallow, medium-sized dish and mix together the paprika, flour, and cayenne. Dip the chicken tenders into this ensuring it is evenly coated.

5. Take a large skillet that is nonstick and pour in 2 teaspoons of olive oil. Place this over medium heat. Make sure the total pan bottom is coated with the oil.

6. Put the chicken into the pan, cook it for about 4 minutes. Flip your chicken and cook for an additional 4 minutes. Repeat this until all chicken tenders are thoroughly cooked.

7. In the same skillet, pour in the rest of the olive oil and allow it to coat the pan's bottom. Add the onion, garlic, and mushrooms. Saute these for about 3 minutes.

8. Remove the pan from the heat.

9. Stir in the mustard and yogurt. Stir until everything is mixed well. Add in the chicken.

10. Serve over the pasta.

Smoky Pork Chops and Tomatoes

This recipe makes 4 servings and takes approximately 35 minutes to make.

Each serving contains:

Protein: 22 grams

Fat: 2.7 grams (0.1 grams saturated fat)

Sodium: 210 milligrams

Cholesterol: 60 milligrams

What's in it

- Diced Roma tomatoes 2 medium
- Canola oil 2 tablespoons
- 5-ounce b1-in pork chops 4
- Black pepper 0.5 teaspoon
- Salt 0.375 teaspoons divided
- Garlic powder 0.25 teaspoons
- Dried thyme leaves 0.5 teaspoons
- Smoked paprika 1 teaspoon
- All-purpose flour 0.25 cups

How it's made

1. Mix the paprika, garlic powder, flour, thyme, pepper and 0.25 teaspoons of salt in a shallow bowl. Evenly coat all pork chops.

2. In a large nonstick pan, pour in the oil and heat it using medium-high heat.

3. Place the pork into the pan and on each side, cook 4 minutes. Repeat until the pork chops are thoroughly cooked.

4. Add in the remaining 0.125 teaspoons of salt and the diced tomatoes. Cook until tomatoes are heated.

CHAPTER 4

DIABETIC-FRIENDLY SNACKS

In between each meal, it is common to get a bit hungry. You want to have a snack, but you have to make sure that it is healthy and diabetic-friendly. There are a number of choices that are easy to prepare, can be stored so that they are always ready to eat, and most importantly, are packed with flavor.

Spinach Yogurt Dip

This recipe makes 24 servings and takes approximately 40 minutes to make.

Each serving contains:

Protein: 2 grams

Fat: 0 grams (0 grams saturated fat)

Sodium: 115 milligrams

Cholesterol: 0 milligrams

What's in it

- Ranch, powdered dressing mix 1 tablespoon

- Chopped, thawed and squeezed spinach 1 cup

- Greek yogurt 1 cup fat-free

- Cottage cheese 1 cup low-fat

How it's made

1. Place the cottage cheese in the blender and puree it.

2. Put the pureed cottage cheese, spinach, yogurt, and dressing powder in a bowl. Thoroughly whisk these together.

3. Place in the refrigerator for 30 minutes to chill it.

Gazpacho Cocktail

This recipe makes 4 servings and takes approximately 10 minutes to make.

Each serving contains:

Protein: 2 grams

Fat: 0 grams (0 grams saturated fat)

Sodium: 300 milligrams

Cholesterol: 0 milligrams

What's in it

- Flat-leaf parsley sprigs 4 large
- Hot pepper sauce 0.25 teaspoons
- Low-sodium tomato juice 1.25 cups
- Clove 1 large
- Prepared horseradish 2 teaspoons
- Vinegar 2 teaspoons Balsamic
- Worcestershire sauce 2 teaspoons vegan
- Lemon juice 1 small
- Chopped scallion 1
- Chopped cucumber 1
- Regular tomato juice 1.25 cups

How it's made

1. Puree the cucumber, juice from the fresh lemon, regular tomato juice, scallion, Worcestershire sauce, horseradish, vinegar, and garlic for about 30 seconds in a blender. Use a low speed. Then, switch to a high speed and puree for an additional 30 seconds.

2. Pour this mixture into a pitcher. Pour in the hot pepper sauce and low-sodium tomato juice. Mix the contents thoroughly and place in the refrigerator until it is time to enjoy. Garnish with a parsley sprig.

Spicy Cream and Baby Carrots Dip

This recipe makes 4 servings and takes approximately 15 minutes to make.

Each serving contains:

Protein: 3 grams

Fat: 2 grams (1 gram saturated fat)

Sodium: 276 milligrams

Cholesterol: 8 milligrams

What's in it

- Baby carrots 48
- Salt 0.25 teaspoon2
- Hot pepper sauce 0.75 teaspoons
- Tub-style, cream cheese 3 tablespoons low-fat
- Sour cream 0.33 cups no-fat

How it's made

1. Grab a large bowl and add the sour cream, pepper sauce, cream cheese, and salt. Mix together until everything is thoroughly blended.

2. Let it sit for 10 minutes so that the flavors develop and serve with the baby carrots.

Spicy and Sweet Whole Grain Mix

This recipe makes 10 servings and takes approximately 40 minutes to make.

Each serving contains:

Protein: 24 grams

Fat: 3 grams (1 gram saturated fat)

Sodium: 216 milligrams

Cholesterol: 0 milligrams

What's in it

- Unsalted, dry-roasted peanuts 0.25 cups
- Unsalted mini pretzels 2 cups
- Wheat cereal squares 2 cups
- Shredded wheat cereal 2 cups
- Ground red pepper 0.25 teaspoons
- Soy sauce 1 tablespoon
- Sugar substitute 0.25 cups
- Egg white 1
- Cooking spray

How it's made

1. At 300 degrees Fahrenheit, preheat the oven.

2. Take a large baking pan that is nonstick and use nonstick spray to evenly coat it.

3. Get a large bowl and put the egg white into it. Whisk this until it becomes foamy. Whisk in the soy sauce, sugar substitute and red pepper.

4. In a medium bowl, mix the pretzels, cereals, and peanuts. Add this to the soy sauce and egg white mixture.

5. Evenly spread this on the baking pan and allow it to cook for 30 minutes. Every 10 minutes, stir the contents.

6. Allow the snack to cool completely before eating.

Garlic-Herb Parmesan Dipping Sticks

This recipe makes 12 servings and takes approximately 40 minutes to make.

Each serving contains:

Protein: 6 grams

Fat: 5 grams (3 grams saturated fat)

Sodium: 404 milligrams

Cholesterol: 11 milligrams

What's in it

- Marinara sauce 1 cup
- Dried oregano 0.5 teaspoons
- Grated Parmesan cheese 0.25 cups
- Italian cheese blend shredded 0.75 cups
- Light herb and garlic spreadable cheese 0.75 cups
- Pre-made pizza dough 13 ounces
- Cooking spray

How it's made

1. At 400 degrees Fahrenheit preheat the oven.
2. Take a medium-sized baking sheet and spray it with cooking spray until it is evenly coated.

3. Roll out the pizza dough onto the baking sheet. Put this into the oven to bake for about 10 minutes.

4. Apply the spreadable cheese evenly using a small spatula. Cover the baked crust with the Parmesan cheese, the Italian cheese blend, and the oregano. Make sure that all of these are sprinkled on evenly. Put this back into the oven for about 15 minutes.

5. Put the marinara sauce into a saucepan. On medium heat, heat this for approximately 8 minutes. Stir frequently to ensure even heating and to maintain the right liquid density.

6. Cut the bread into 8 rows lengthwise. Cut it again along the width into the 3 rows. Serve up on a platter with the heated marinara sauce.

Mediterranean Tuna Cups

This recipe makes 10 servings and takes approximately 15 minutes to make.

Each serving contains:

Protein: 5 grams

Fat: 1 gram (0 grams saturated fat)

Sodium: 102 milligrams

Cholesterol: 8 milligrams

What's in it

- White albacore tuna in water, flaked and drained 10 ounces

- Garlic salt 0.25 teaspoons

- Lemon juice 2 tablespoons fresh

- Red onion 0.33 cups chopped

- Pitted and chopped Kalamata olives 0.33 cups

- Non-fat, plain Greek yogurt 0.66 cups

- Cucumbers 3 medium

How it's made

1. Slice each cucumber into 10 pieces, discarding the ends. Keep the cucumber shell and use a 0.5 teaspoon to scoop out the insides. Make sure that there is a thin

layer on the bottom of each slice so that it can accommodate the tuna mixture.

2. Stir together the olives, garlic, yogurt, onion and lemon juice. Blend until the mixture is smooth. Add in the tuna and stir again until it is all blended.

3. Take approximately 1 tablespoon of the tuna mix and put it into the cucumber cup. Repeat this until all 10 of the cucumber cups are filled with tuna. Keep this refrigerated until eating.

CHAPTER 5

DIABETIC-FRIENDLY DESSERT OPTIONS

When you get a sweet tooth, there is nothing wrong with indulging as long as you make the right choices. As a diabetic, not any sweet treat will do. However, this does not mean that you have to completely shy away from your favorites. There are several dessert options that are not only decadent, but you can eat them completely guilt-free too.

Sweet Peanut Butter Dip

This recipe makes 4 servings and takes approximately 10 minutes to make.

Each serving contains:

Protein: 3 grams

Fat: 1 gram (1 gram saturated fat)

Sodium: 51 milligrams

Cholesterol: 0 milligrams

What's in it

- Sliced banana 2 medium

- Packed dark brown sugar 2 teaspoons

- Reduced-fat peanut butter 2 tablespoons

- Vanilla, fat-free yogurt 0.33 cups

How it's made

1. Place the peanut butter, yogurt and brown sugar in a bowl. Whisk together until completely mixed.

2. Place the bananas on top of the peanut butter mixture.

Rainbow Shishkabob

This recipe makes 25 servings and takes approximately 20 minutes to make.

Each serving contains:

Protein: 2 grams

Fat: 0.5 grams (0.1 grams saturated fat)

Sodium: 10 milligrams

Cholesterol: 0 milligrams

What's in it

- Blackberries 3 cups
- Purple grapes 3 cups
- Blueberries 4 cups
- Green grapes 3 cups
- Cored, cubed and peeled pineapple 1 whole
- Cubed cantaloupe 4 cups
- Hulled strawberries 4 cups
- Cinnamon 0.125 teaspoons
- Chia seeds 1 tablespoon
- 100-calorie, vanilla Greek yogurt 8 ounces

How it's made

1. Mix together the chia seeds, yogurt and cinnamon to make the dipping sauce.

2. Using a skewering stick, place 1 of each fruit onto it. Use the same order for all 25 sticks.

3. Serve on a platter with the dipping sauce.

Maple and Cinnamon Peaches

This recipe makes 4 servings and takes approximately 15 minutes to make.

Each serving contains:

Protein: 1 gram

Fat: 0 grams (0.1 grams saturated fat)

Sodium: 0 milligrams

Cholesterol: 0 milligrams

What's in it

- Maple syrup 1 tablespoon
- Nutmeg 0.125 teaspoons
- Cinnamon 0.5 teaspoons
- Lemon juice 1 medium
- Ripe peaches 4

How it's made

1. Preheat the grill until it gets to medium-high heat.

2. Mix the nutmeg, maple syrup, lemon juice and cinnamon. Roll the peaches until they are fully and evenly coated.

3. Grill the peaches for approximately 4 minutes until golden brown. Turn them once.

Peanut Butter Swirl Chocolate Brownies

This recipe makes 20 servings and takes approximately 40 minutes to make.

Each serving contains:

Protein: 3 grams

Fat: 8 grams (3 grams saturated fat)

Sodium: 61 milligrams

Cholesterol: 6 milligrams

What's in it

- Mini semisweet chocolate chips 0.25 cups
- Unsweetened cocoa powder 0.5 cups
- Creamy low-fat peanut butter 0.25 cups
- Baking powder 1 teaspoon
- All-purpose flour 1.25 cups
- Vanilla 1 teaspoon
- Canola oil 0.25 cups
- Egg substitute 0.75 cups
- Cold water 0.33 cups
- Granulated sugar 0.66 cups
- Butter 0.25 cups

53

- Cooking spray

How it's made

1. At 350 degrees Fahrenheit, preheat the oven.

2. Take a baking pan that measures 9x9x2 and coat it with foil, ensuring the total bottom and sides are covered.

3. Use a nonstick spray for fully coat the foil.

4. Grab a medium-sized saucepan, place it on a low heat and melt the butter. Take the pan off of the heat and whisk in the water and sugar. Stir in the oil, vanilla, and egg. Whisk until fully mixed. Pour in the baking powder and flour and mix completely.

5. In a bowl, pour in the peanut butter. Slowly whisk in 0.5 cups of the butter and flour mixture.

6. Grab a separate small bowl and combine the cocoa powder and 0.25 cups of flour. Stir in the chocolate chips and plain batter. Pour this mixture into the pan that was prepared earlier.

7. On top of the chocolate batter, put the peanut butter mixture. Swirl the 2 together using a thin spatula. Metal works best.

8. Once swirled, place in the oven and bake for 20 to 25 minutes.

Coconut Cream Pie

This recipe makes 10 servings and takes approximately 40 minutes to make.

Each serving contains:

Protein: 7 grams

Fat: 10 grams (4 grams saturated fat)

Sodium: 147 milligrams

Cholesterol: 66 milligrams

What's in it

- Cold water 5 tablespoons
- Shortening 0.33 cups
- Salt 0.25 teaspoons
- All-purpose flour 1.25 cups
- Flaked coconut 2 tablespoons
- Sugar 0.33 cups
- Cream of tartar 0.25 teaspoons
- Vanilla 0.5 teaspoons
- Coconut extract 1 teaspoon
- Fat-free evaporated milk 12 ounces
- Fat-free milk 1.5 coups

- Cornstarch 0.25 cups

- Sugar 0.25 cups

- Whole eggs 3

How it's made

1. Separate the whites from the yolks and put the whites in 1 bowl and the yolks in another.

2. Take a medium saucepan and combine the cornstarch and 0.25 cups of sugar. Gradually mix in the evaporated and regular milk. Over medium heat, cook until thick. Remove from heat and add the beaten egg yolks. Get this boiling and then reduce the heat. Cook for an additional 2 minutes.

3. Mix in the coconut extract and take the pan from the stove to stir. This completes the pie filling.

4. Take the egg white bowl and add the cream of tartar and vanilla. Using medium speed on a mixer, beat this together for approximately 30 seconds. Add in the 0.33 cups of sugar and beat at high speed. Only add 1 tablespoon at a time. Once it is all in, beat for 2 more minutes. This is the meringue.

5. Create the pie shell. Mix together the salt and flour. Cut the shortening into pea-sized portions. Using 1 tablespoon at a time, sprinkle the water onto the salt and flour mixture. Add in the shortening. Mix until all ingredients are used, and there is a ball of pastry.

6. Spread the shell ball out on a pie pan that is about 9 inches around.

7. Pour the pie filling part into the shell. Spread it evenly and then put the meringue right on top. Make sure that

the edges are sealed. Sprinkle the coconut flakes on top of this.

8. Preheat the oven to 350 degrees Fahrenheit. Once heated, put the pie in the oven for approximately 15 minutes. Let it cool before serving.

CONCLUSION

Thank you for making it through to the end of this book, let's hope it was informative and able to provide you with all of the tools you need to achieve your goals whatever they may be.

The next step is to take note of the recipes that you want to try first. Head to the store and grab the ingredients so that you are ready to enjoy indulgent meals that are healthy and ideal for the diabetic lifestyle. All of these recipes include ingredients that are easy to find and preparation steps that are quick and simple. This means that you can start enjoying these delicious recipes today.

Finally, if you found this book useful in any way, a review on Amazon is always appreciated!

Lightning Source UK Ltd.
Milton Keynes UK
UKHW012050170221
378966UK00003B/366